21st April

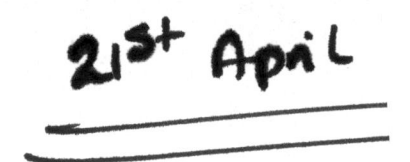

The DIY Spa Retreat

Design A Resort-Style Retreat At Home

By Heather R. Tremko

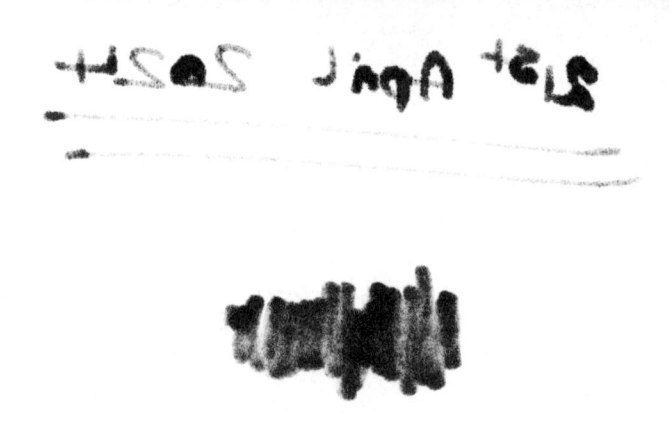

Copyright © 2015 Heather R. Tremko

ALL RIGHTS RESERVED. No part of this publication may be reproduced or transmitted in any form whatsoever, electronic, or mechanical, including photocopying, recording, or by any informational storage or retrieval system without express written, dated and signed permission from the author.

ISBN: 1523364173
ISBN-13: 978-1523364176

CONTENTS

1	How to use this book	4
2	Introduction	6
3	Preparatory Steps	10
4	Beauty Treatments	13
5	Stretches, Yoga, Pilates	17
6	Spa Meals	19
7	Meditations and Affirmations	24
8	Workshops and Journaling	26
9	Entertainment	31
10	Sleep	34
11	Wrapping it all up	37
12	Appendix: Sample Schedules	38
13	Appendix: Meal Recipes	42
14	Appendix: Affirmations	47
15	Appendix: Spa Music	48
16	30 Ideas for a Couples Retreat	49

HOW TO USE THIS BOOK

In this book you will find chapters covering the following topics: beauty treatments, physical exercises, meditation and affirmation, personal growth workshops and journaling, recipes for spa meals and beverages, ideas for entertainment outside of your home or hotel room, and guidance on getting a good night's sleep. Each chapter lists sources and ideas to inspire you, but **the chapters are by no means exhaustive. Otherwise, each section would end up being a book all by itself.** Think of each section as being a curated list of techniques, so you don't have to waste your own time Googling everything from scratch.

Read the book straight through, or just skip to the topics that interest you. There are probably more ideas here than you can fit into a one or two-day retreat. Some of the ideas are contradictory. For example, depending on the type of retreat you are designing, you may choose to have no screen time, or you might want to binge-watch a favorite show. Not all of the suggestions are going to work for every reader. Pick and choose events that you like, creating a custom spa schedule for yourself.

The DIY Spa Retreat is meant to be a personal planning retreat for one person. However, most of the suggested activities would easily adapt to a couple's retreat. At the end of the book, I list 30 additional ideas ideal for a couple's retreat.

I love collecting information for the DIY Spa Retreat and periodically I find new sources that would be perfect for the book. If you would like to receive the periodic newsletter with new sources, you can email me directly at DIYSpaRetreat@gmail.com to let me know. Also feel free to email me if you have any questions about the sources, or need a pdf file for easier reading, or for any reason at all!

INTRODUCTION

It got to the point where I had to throw all my travel magazines away. Do you know this feeling? I spent far too much of my time browsing through the pages of travel brochures, and I had to figure out how to stop daydreaming and start living in the real world. *My* real world. I could achieve my ideal retreat without making it a once-in-a-lifetime expense.

We all have our own ideas of what makes the perfect luxurious retreat. Personally I would opt for a world-class hotel, with private spa facilities and a rooftop infinity pool overlooking stunning mountain views, where I could watch the sun go down while sipping on an ice cold spritzer. The advertisements for spa resorts sell a dream that, for the majority of us, is out of reach. Thousands of miles away from home and at a price most of us would need a lottery win to afford. And even if money were no object, it simply isn't always possible to rearrange your life to make the dream a reality. But once in a while we all need to relax and recharge the batteries. And if a villa in Dubai is out of the question, then for our own sanity and well-being we must find an affordable, alternative solution closer to home.

I wholeheartedly believe that self-care should not be seen as a luxury. Self-care is a right, and something we often deny ourselves. We've all heard the often-repeated metaphor that when the flight attendant directs us to put on our own masks before assisting others, this is just a metaphor for self-care in everyday life. You cannot care for others if you do not take time to care for yourself. Each day we find the time to shower and brush our teeth, but rarely do we place the same level of importance on our mental health.

Most people find when they are properly rested (both mentally and physically), they are able to deal with everyday tasks more efficiently. They are less likely to lose their tempers, make silly mistakes, or forget important information.

Taking a break is nothing to be ashamed of and certainly nothing to feel guilty about. If the idea of taking a break causes you stress, ask yourself why? Are you putting pressure on yourself (or the vacation) to make everything perfect? It does not have to be perfect. Consider scheduling small retreats for yourself on a regular basis – twice a year, or quarterly. Does taking a vacation make you feel guilty? You don't need to prove to anyone that you are a hard worker, especially by not taking time off. You deserve to relax. You *need* to relax. By working hard you are setting a fantastic example for your children/roommates/significant other/co-workers/boss, but they also need to understand that "me time" is an important part of a balanced and happy life.

Let me be clear. The term "self-care" extends beyond physical care such as pedicures and massages. I'm referring to a bigger picture that includes being kind to ourselves, not demanding perfection, allowing ourselves to say no, letting go of guilt, and giving ourselves rest and downtime.

Many great thinkers are famous for taking private retreats. Bill Gates is known for taking a "think week" twice each year. Family, friends, and employees are banned. He says, "By actively disconnecting ... I am able to effectively reflect, reset, and clearly rethink my goals and aspirations ... I create a life to-do list, do a lot of research, and think through big ideas and challenges deeply. Going through this process has been enlightening."

Although no one else can claim the resources that Bill Gates has, I still suggest that even the busiest among us can carve out some time to reflect and reset as well. The payoffs will be worth the investment of your time.

Self-care is not something that most of us were taught, so it may feel unnatural or selfish. When people are asked why they don't take time for themselves, here are the common answers. *I'm too crazy-busy. There aren't enough hours in the day. Breaks are for the weak. I'll sleep when I'm dead. My kids cry when I leave. My partner makes me feel guilty. My boss makes me feel guilty.* Also because self-care is not commonly taught, you may get resistance from those around you. You know when you need to take some time out. You will need to be firm with yourself and those around you - there is no need to feel guilty or ashamed.

If at this time you are already thinking "yeah right, I really DON'T have the time for this," then do give me a chance and read on. You will see that even if you can only carve out ten minutes, that there are plenty of resources here that will help you see those ten minutes as if you were in a spa.

So is it possible to recreate the luxury spa retreat experience? I believe it is! I looked at several spa retreat schedules and realized that a similar experience could easily be created either in my home, or in a local hotel of my own choosing, at a fraction of the cost of a luxury spa retreat. I do understand that when I am running my own retreat "staycation", the sense of being waited on is going to be missing. But I will gain the recharging and relaxation that was my ultimate goal anyway. I save money by not having a personal chef, beautician, yoga instructor, meditation guide, counselor, workshop educator, hiking leader, and concierge. Instead I will seek out local experts or utilize free or low-cost media tools available to me via websites, podcasts, YouTube, phone/tablet apps, and print books or audiobooks (either purchased or via library loans).

The aim of this book is to show you that with a bit of imagination and a few minor compromises, it is most definitely possible to plan your own resort-style retreat at home. Best of all, the benefits of your home retreat will come from your intentions, not from how much money you spend.

Here is a sample schedule for one of my spa retreat staycations. (There are many more sample schedules in the Appendix, including the 2-day retreat, the holiday planning retreat, the beach day, and the distraction retreat.) This one was a single-day retreat during which my husband took our children out of the house for the day. The purpose of the retreat was to have some personal quiet time, and also to review goals that I had made several months prior.

***

Morning: Wake and do a morning stretch as guided by a YouTube video on my tablet. Bathe and do a full-body scrub using a homemade sugar scrub. Have a healthy spa breakfast in my own kitchen, using fresh produce that I purchased the day before. Give myself a manicure and pedicure while listening to music of my own choosing (not my children's choosing!). I enjoy a steam facial using a vaporizer/humidifier. I color my hair. Do a guided meditation using a favorite phone app.

Late Morning/Early Afternoon: Head outdoors for a nature hike. Then prepare and eat a healthy spa lunch in my own kitchen.

Afternoon: Journaling. Review my previously written goals and check in with myself to see how those goals are progressing. Then I identify a goal upon which I can take some immediate action, and use the next two hours to make progress on that goal. (Though I don't want to get too specific about my personal goals, examples are things like: work on my family's online photo album, work on an unfinished hobby project, or complete an activity that helps our family business move forward.)

Evening: Have dinner. I've decided to go out and enjoy a prepared meal at a local farm-to-table restaurant. Enjoy evening entertainment. A local art museum has an "after dark" event, and I attend and enjoy the art with a glass of wine.

***

PREPARATORY STEPS

DETERMINE YOUR REASON FOR THE RETREAT

What is your reason for taking this spa retreat? How do you want to feel at the close of the retreat? It's hard to choose a path when you don't have a destination in mind. Here are some common reasons:

- I simply want a fun weekend to relax and recharge.

- I need to focus on a difficult decision.

- I need a temporary escape from something going on in my everyday life.

- I am taking a regularly scheduled retreat to check in on my goals and resolutions.

- I need to take time for discovery, self-improvement, or a whole life audit.

Knowing your goal will help you to design an event that works for you.

DETERMINE THE LOCATION AND DATE OF YOUR RETREAT

Once you have determined your personal reasons for needing a spa retreat, the next step is to decide on the date and location. Make it a priority to clear your schedule for one or two days. If this is utterly impossible, then choose a time when you can block out a couple of hours in the morning or evening. Or, if you only have ten minutes, then **embrace that, and start with ten minutes**. You will find plenty of activities in this book that are suitable for a ten-minute timeout for yourself.

Will you conduct your retreat in your own home, or would a local hotel room be a better fit for you? Or maybe you'd like an unconventional location for your retreat. Each location has pros and cons.

Retreat at home: The biggest drawback to staying home is that it might not provide a feeling of escape. Our homes are often full of visual clutter, reminders of to-do lists, and people who may cause us stress through their noises or presence. External noise can severely limit your focus, relaxation, and the ability to hear your inner voice. There are workarounds for some of these problems, which I will address later. Otherwise, the home staycation is more frugal and convenient than a hotel room. And at least one informal study that I read indicated that mothers especially appreciate the rarity of being alone in their own homes. If you can resist the urge to do housework, then you might ask your partner or a friend to take the kids out of the house for several hours or overnight.

Retreat at a local hotel: A hotel room can be wonderfully refreshing and need not be too pricey. But, depending on how you've customized your retreat events, you may have a lot of inconvenient packing and unpacking to do. For example, if you've scheduled a lot of beauty treatments, you'll have to bring them with you to the hotel. If you're just bringing a journal and smartphone, this isn't such an issue.

Retreat at a friend's home: Can a friend loan you a room for your retreat? Or maybe you and a friend would like to trade homes for a weekend. Decide if this would help you focus on your goals, or if it would just be distracting.

Short and sweet retreat at a city park: If you only have a day, pare the retreat down to the minimum required "stuff" and drive to a park. Maybe one you've never been to before. Pack your lunch, or go to a deli or natural foods store and grab stuff for a picnic.

BEFORE THE RETREAT BEGINS

After you've decided on the date and location of your staycation, sketch out a schedule of events for the retreat. It need not be a static schedule. Feel free to break the rules and change it up during the actual event. The only reason you need an idea of a schedule now is so that you know what kind of preparatory work you will need to do before your staycation. During the actual retreat, I want you to act on inspiration.

Let everyone close to you know that you will not be available during your retreat. If you can, you will turn on your out-of-office reply on your email and text, and put your phone on "do not disturb" mode.

Preview any media that you plan to use during your retreat. Download apps.

Review your custom schedule, and shop for any special items you want for your staycation. Get your groceries and ingredients for any beauty treatments that you want to make.

If you are staying home ...

• Declutter the space where you will be spending the most time. Bedroom and bathroom? Writing area? Take some time to really clean up those spaces so you can better achieve relaxation and focus. Hotel rooms tend to be relaxing because they lack the day-to-day visual clutter that we have at home. If it isn't feasible to permanently deal with your visual clutter, see if you can at least temporarily hide it – in a box, behind a curtain, something like that.

• Get rid of the junk food. Imagine you are the chef at a world-class spa. Clean out your fridge and cupboards and remove all the things you would not dream of serving to spa guests. You are going to shop for meals that are both delicious and beneficial.

• Can you make arrangements to send the kids to Grandma's for the weekend?

If you are going to a hotel ...

• Make your hotel reservation. Choose a hotel that has the amenities that are important to you and will benefit you during your retreat. For example, if you plan to prepare meals in your room, you'll want to reserve a room with a kitchenette. If you don't plan to cook or if the room does not have a kitchenette, see if they have a restaurant on-site, or if there are delivery options nearby. If you want to soak in a bathtub, make sure the room actually has a bathtub and that it is a decent size. Try to avoid hotels in locations that will cause you frustration due to traffic or lack of parking.

• Consider making your selected beauty treatments in advance so you do not have to pack excess ingredients. Same goes for your spa meals ... some can be prepared in advance as well.

BEAUTY TREATMENTS

This chapter is probably the lightest in tone, but it's fun and contains some of the more common items that women love to schedule into a spa retreat. I like to start my staycations with some beauty treatments, because I'm much more comfortable and able to relax when I feel more presentable and pulled together. The way a good hair day affects your attitude all day, let these self-care ideas set the tone for your retreat. I've tried to recommend treatments that are not too harsh and that avoid common allergens. If you have specific recipes you've saved on your Pinterest board to "try later," now's the time.

• Prepare a simple white sugar scrub using only 2 ingredients from your kitchen. 1 cup of white sugar combined with ½ cup of oil makes a wonderful scrub for hands, elbows, heels, or décolletage when used at the end of a shower or bath. Grapeseed oil is great for skin but, really, you can use any cooking oil you have in the kitchen. If you have essential oils, go ahead and add several drops of whatever fragrance you like.

• Or try a brown sugar scrub. Combine 1 cup brown sugar with 1/3 cup olive oil (or oil of your choice). Use immediately, or store in a glass jar for later use.

• Give yourself a proper manicure. Take the time to soak your fingertips in a bowl or sink of warm water for a few minutes. Treat your cuticles, and then use a hand moisturizer and allow it to penetrate for half an hour. Use a base coat, color, and top coat. My manicure hack is to use a clear polish containing glitter for my main color. My fingernails look polished, but as long as it's a glitter floating in a clear base, any chips appear invisible and my manicure appears to last longer. If you aren't sure how to give yourself a manicure, there's great how-to article at TinyURL.com/WikiManicure.

• Try a steam facial. This feels really luxurious if you are doing your spa staycation during cold winter months. Make sure your face is clean and makeup removed before you begin. You can do the old-fashioned method of boiling water and pouring it into a large bowl, then draping a towel over your head as you breathe the steam. I like using a room humidifier for longer-lasting steam. I use the Vicks 1.5 gallon steam vaporizer, designed for use in children's nurseries. You can add herbal teabags and/or essential oils to the water for more of a spa experience. Tea tree and eucalyptus oils are anti-bacterial, so these are nice for skin, but any essential oils are a treat.

• Apply a facial mask after you steam your face (or if you choose not to steam, put a wet warm washcloth on your face for a few minutes first). Oatmeal masks have an excellent safety record and are highly moisturizing. Oatmeal masks can be used on all skin types, even sensitive skin. You can use whole oats, or grind them into a powder (a.k.a. *colloidal oats*), then cook a small serving as directed on the package, with either water or milk. Once it has cooled to a comfortable temperature, apply to your face with very clean hands. Lie down and let the mask do its work for at least 10 minutes, then wipe off with a washcloth, and rinse your face with water.

• Not into DIY masks? Your local drugstore should have some single-application clay masks or peel-off masks for a reasonable price.

• Follow a mask treatment with a simple facial toner made from 1 part apple cider vinegar to 4 parts water.

• Hair likes to have a mask too. Coconut oil is known to penetrate the actual hair follicle and has been confirmed to lead to less hair breakage when used regularly. You can apply it as an overnight mask, or make your own hot oil treatment. Warm the oil in the microwave and then apply to your hair, pop on a shower cap, and wait at least 15 minutes before shampooing it out. If you have a plastic squeeze bottle (like the kind that comes with home hair color kits), it will come in handy.

• Take a bath. Any kind of bath that you like. This is purely psychological, so whether you prefer bubbles, Epsom salt, oatmeal baths, or just a long soak – enjoy and relax.

• If you feel like spending money, head out of your cocoon to indulge in some paid treatments. Book a massage or a hair wash and style. Or head to the beauty counter for a makeover or makeup lesson. Check reviews online before deciding on a service.

STRETCHES, YOGA, PILATES

Virtually every spa offers a variety of exercise classes, with the most common being some type of yoga. A really cool thing about a destination spa is that the spa is typically located in a beautiful nature setting, such as the beach, or the red rocks of Utah or Arizona. These spas offer outdoor exercise classes, so you can stretch or do yoga while being inspired by the beautiful nature around you.

If you happen to live near a place where you can practice yoga in nature, give it a try. A beach, a park, or even your backyard are great options for this.

But, if it's winter or you just don't have access to a beautiful outdoor setting, you can at least try YouTube for inspiration. Of course this will be nothing like practicing yoga at Red Rocks, but has its own advantages. Have fun with it. If you're inexperienced and need some ideas, here are some YouTube links to try out. Most of the videos are very short, so if you're having fun, do two or more.

• *Beginner yoga at the beach*. This 7-minute video really makes me smile, and I think you won't be able to help smiling either. It's filmed on a city beach, and the gal who leads it is a beginner herself. There is nothing intimidating about the instructor or this brief yoga stretch. If you want to start your day with some simple yoga, this one will make you happy. The exact link is: https://youtu.be/BT8gsb2O9ww, or go to YouTube channel JaaackJack, click on the little magnifying glass to open the Search box, and type in "Beach Yoga".

• *Stretch/yoga at the beach*. Compared to the previous video, this 9-minute video is filmed closer to the water. The instructor has more of a cheerleader tone about her, but she is friendly and motivating. Exact link: https://youtu.be/Qgz4o2lEXYQ, or go to YouTube channel blogilates and search for "Relax with me" on her channel.

• *Rodney Yee* beginner *yoga at the beach*. A 5 ½ minute yoga stretch beautifully filmed on Molokai. Exact link: https://youtu.be/NMYSRCCLeGw, or go to YouTube channel Gaiam and search for "Yoga for beginners morning".

• *Yoga at Red Rocks*. The female instructor does a lovely job in this 11-minute video, and gets into some more meditative poses than the previous videos do. Exact link: https://youtu.be/UelBL9VD3Zc. Her channel does not have a search feature, but from YouTube's main page you can search for "Sania Shakti Yoga Red Rock".

• *Mini-workout for the waist*. This video is led by Miranda Esmonde-White of PBS. It's under 4 ½ minutes and is filmed at a resort in Jamaica. The exact link is way too long to print, but you can find the video by going to YouTube and searching on the name of the video: "Classical Stretch mini workout to slenderize waist."

• *Classical Stretch in Jamaica*. Here is an 8-minute stretch filmed at Montego Bay. You'll need a chair for this one. The instructor starts the video by saying it's a 5-minute stretch, but it's really about 8 minutes. The YouTube channel is Essentrics Workout, and the name of the video is "Essentrics Stretch at Iberostar."

• *Beginner Pilates*. This is a full workout (28 minutes) filmed in a park – I'm not sure exactly where. Instructor Kim Wilson has gotten great reviews on this Pilates workout. Exact link: https://youtu.be/To8PByzhtTw, or go to YouTube channel DoYogaWithMe and search for "Pilates: Beginner".

SPA MEALS

It goes without saying (but I'll say it anyway) that your spa retreat menu can be whatever you like. If you want to spend your staycation eating nothing but cake, that is your prerogative. However, one of the draws of the spa resort is that they are able to provide an amazing menu of healthy and delicious meals. I am assuming that most readers are at least a little bit interested in replicating this type of menu during a home spa day.

In this chapter you will find ideas for single-serving meals that can easily be prepared at home or in a hotel kitchenette. I avoid complex meals that take all day to cook, meals that don't travel well, and meals with unusual ingredients that I might not use up later. Although this eliminates many meals commonly served at famous spa resorts, there still remain many delicious meals that adapt well to the spa staycation. And of course you can still choose to prepare a more complicated meal, or go out to a restaurant. When I treat myself to an at-home spa weekend, I typically go out for at least one dinner.

If you have zero experience with cooking, you probably don't want to start during your spa weekend and end up stressing yourself out. But you can get some ideas for purchased meals that add to the tone of your staycation.

BREAKFAST

- Granola cereals are high in fiber and are very satisfying, so that a little goes a long way. When you're shopping at your local grocery store, read the ingredient labels on the granola cereals before making your choice. You'll see that not all granola cereals are created equal – they vary widely in the amount and type of sweeteners used. If you have time, you can make your own granola cereal in advance of your spa staycation. See the Appendix for a great recipe for homemade granola.

• Scramble eggs with some greens and herbs for a nourishing and beautiful spa breakfast. Chop some fresh spinach or kale, and then heat with some butter or oil in a skillet until the leaves are wilted (about a minute). Whisk 2 eggs with some thyme, parsley, or oregano (fresh, if you can). Add the egg mixture to the skillet and scramble as usual.

• Crepes with mascarpone (or ricotta, or cottage cheese) and fresh fruit – a real treat for me – and I take the shortcut and use store-bought crepes, found in the produce section in the grocery store. Most recipes for homemade crepes require that the batter be left to set for 30 minutes to an hour. I personally don't care to wait that long when we're talking about breakfast. I warm the store-bought crepe a little, using the microwave. Then add a bit of mascarpone and roll it up, and top with fresh fruit. You can macerate the fruit in a little bit of sugar if you like.

LUNCH

• Asian slaw – I love, love, love this salad. I often make it in big batches and take it to potlucks and there are never any leftovers. The vinegar dressing gives it some bite, which is offset by the sugar. Feel free to scale back on the sugar, or substitute with another sweetener. This recipe serves more than one person, but if you are traveling to a hotel you can assemble the salad in advance and just bring a single-serving portion with you. The main ingredients are a cabbage slaw or broccoli slaw base, to which you may add chopped apples, green onions, and cooked chicken (if you prefer). See the Appendix for the complete recipe.

• One of my favorite lunches is a grilled Caprese sandwich. This vegetarian meal only has five ingredients, all of which are fresh, real food, and it's on my plate in under 10 minutes. See the Appendix for the complete recipe.

- Mason jar salads are trendy now, and they are ideal for your retreat because they can be made in single servings and are easily portable. Make it special by choosing ingredients in a variety of colors, and then layering them. It's a fun way to "eat the rainbow". Try special ingredients that you don't normally put in your daily salads. Radishes or pomegranate seeds for red. Mandarin oranges. Cheeses. Quinoa. Red onions. You can make a layered pasta salad the same way.

DINNER

- Salmon is a staple at spa resorts. It's generally accepted to be a superfood, due to its high quantity of omega-3 fatty acids. And it's delicious and easy to prepare. You can purchase single servings of salmon at your grocery store, either fresh or frozen. Do yourself a favor and make sure it's been de-boned first. My favorite method of cooking salmon is to put onto a big square of foil, and then put some Italian salad dressing on top. Wrap it up in a foil square and then put in the fridge to marinate. If you forget to marinate it in advance, don't worry about it. Even 20 minutes while you are pre-heating the oven or grill is fine. If you are grilling, cook the foil packet about 3-5 minutes on each side. If you are baking, cook the foil packet in a 350-degree oven for about 20 minutes (I start checking the fish at 10 minutes, and again at 15 minutes). When the fish flakes easily with a fork, it's done. Serve with veggies or your favorite side dish.

- Another high protein meal is the Tex-Mex pork chop. Start with a boneless pork chop or pork tenderloins. Season the raw meat with some packaged fajita seasoning, or whatever seasoning you like. Heat some butter or olive oil in a skillet over medium heat, then sauté the pork on each side. About 2 minutes per side for a thin (1/2 inch) chop, or up to 6 minutes per side for a thicker (1.5 inch) chop. Remove the pork chop to your dinner plate. Then mix equal parts heavy cream and salsa, and add to the skillet. Bring to a boil, then simmer for a couple of minutes, stirring constantly. Pour the sauce over your pork chop. Serve with your favorite side dish.

- I only recently learned about zucchini noodles, which are just noodles that you've cut from a zuke using a potato peeler or a mandolin. These versatile noodles can be served raw, or lightly stir-fried (cook for about one minute). Top the noodles with anything you would normally serve with pasta. Chopped tomatoes with garlic, Alfredo sauce, parmesan, basil, anything.

BEVERAGES

- Spa water! Spa water is all the rage right now. I feel like I could (jokingly) tell you that *you can't truly have a spa experience if you don't have spa water.* It is sort of funny as to how much attention spa water is getting. I even got caught up in the fun of it, and I bought a special infused water pitcher (which isn't necessary, by the way). So here goes. Spa water is water that has been infused with fruit, vegetables, or spices. There are 2 types of infused waters. One type of water has cut fruit, etc. floating in the water, and the water itself remains virtually clear. The other type is where the fruit, etc. is muddled into the water, creating what is effectively a very watery smoothie. See the Appendix for ideas for both types of infused waters.

- Speaking of smoothies ... I feel almost sorry for smoothies, having now been upstaged by spa water. Nevertheless, smoothies are delicious and healthy, and can even serve as meal replacements during your spa day. Here's a general formula for creating your own smoothie. Start with a very soft fruit like a banana, avocado, peach, or mango. Add one cup of berries or other fruit. Then add about three tablespoons of fat, like almonds or coconut milk. Add a little protein powder, cottage cheese, or yogurt. Then add a cup of liquid, like water, nut milk, or juice. Top off with three ice cubes, and blend. If you used any frozen fruit, you can skip the ice cubes. If the smoothie is too thick, add some more liquid. If it's too thin, add some more fruit or ice cubes.

MEDITATIONS AND AFFIRMATIONS

I viewed dozens of spa resort websites to check out the activities they offered. Nearly every resort offered meditation classes or guided meditations. Many people view this activity as a necessary element of a wellness retreat. Once you become experienced, you may well view this activity as a necessary element of daily life. If you are already experienced in meditation, skip ahead to the bulleted list of sources. If you're not experienced, read on.

Meditation is known to improve both mental and physical health. It is for everyone and all types of people and personalities. You don't have to join a group or believe in anything. It is secular, and scientifically validated.

To the non-practitioner, the most common belief about meditation is that it is difficult. Both fictional characters in books and film, and real-life journalists and media personalities, commonly report a brief dalliance with meditation as being "the hardest thing I've ever done" ... "I was dripping with sweat at the exertion of forcing myself to do nothing." This is unfortunate negative press, created by people who are complicating a very simple concept. The hardest thing about meditation is comprehending how easy it actually is.

Yes, there are various practices in meditation that may be considered to be advanced. We don't need to address these during our retreats. We don't need to spend our spa time learning about theta waves or attempting Vipassana meditation. There are as many types of meditation as there are diets. You may only be somewhat familiar with Zen meditation, conjuring up an image of the person sitting with a straight back, desperately trying to not have a thought. That is only one of many forms, so be aware that there are numerous other forms of meditation.

Yes, your mind will wander. Your brain is a chatterbox. That's what it is wired to be. It is normal — in fact, if you are able to shut off any thoughts, you probably need to be hospitalized. And that is why spas offer guided meditations, so you can listen to a coach who gives you words, memories, or feelings on which to focus.

All of the recommended sources are free and do not require a login.

• My first recommendation is the Omvana app, available for both iPhone and Android platforms. When you open the app, you will be offered the chance to create an account, but it is not mandatory. The free app comes with guided meditations. Additional meditations for specific subjects (such as weight loss, finding love, and overcoming insomnia) are available for purchase. If they don't automatically download, search for these 3 meditations by Vishen Lakhiani: *Beginners Meditation Day 1* (8 minutes), *Beginners Meditation Day 2* (9 minutes), and the *6 Phase Meditation* (20 minutes). You can listen to the "Day 1" and "Day 2" tutorials back-to-back in one session. They don't literally need to be a day apart. The 6-phase meditation covers general focus, relaxation, and gratitude, and Vishen assumes you are doing it first thing in the morning, but really you can play it any time.

• If you prefer a female voice, try the Calm app, available in both IOS and Android platforms. Like Omvana, when you open the app, you will be offered a chance to log in but you can skip that. Calm combines tutorial with actual meditation practice. If you don't want the tutorials, click on "Guided" at the top of the screen to access free guided meditations. The meditations range from 3 minutes to 25 minutes in length, with the same female voice used in the tutorials.

• You can also use Calm without downloading an app. Open the website www.calm.com, and you have instant access to free guided meditations from 2 to 20 minutes in length. These are guided by a female voice, but it is a different voice from the one used on the Calm app. The meditations are very easy to follow, but if you feel you need more basic training, Calm also has a series of 7 instructional videos that are available at TinyURL.com/CalmTraining. These videos are led by the same female voice used on the website.

• Definitely check out the YouTube channel by TheHonestGuys. These guys are awesome! There are so many wonderful videos, which you don't really need to watch – just listen. The guided meditations are so relaxing and easy to listen to. You aren't tasked with thinking about anything. It's more like listening to a story. In fact, they have some that really are stories where you imagine yourself visiting Tolkien's Middle Earth. The geek inside you will love it.

• If you prefer meditating without voice guidance, try playing some nature sounds or spa music while focusing on your breath, or repeating an affirmation that resonates with you. I have an affirmation that my first-grade teacher made us repeat daily, and it's still stuck in my head. *Every day in every way, I am getting better, better, and better. I am a happy, healthy person.* She added a melody and had us sing it each morning. I still use it to bring my mind to focus. See the Appendix for more suggested affirmations.

WORKSHOPS AND JOURNALING

The famous world-class spa resorts frequently offer self-improvement classes or workshops. As I write this, Miraval Resort is offering five classes to their spa guests, with fees averaging $60-$100 per hour, and titles ranging from "mastering your makeup" to "life is simple." Red Mountain Resort in Utah offers private life coaching sessions as well as several classes ranging from photography to "mindful eating." Sunrise Springs in New Mexico offers "therapeutic gardening" and stress consultations. "Zendoodle" and "journaling for self-discovery" are two of the many classes offered at The Lodge at Woodloch in the Poconos.

At your spa retreat, you can customize your own workshop. You can seek out teachers via YouTube or podcasts or library books. You can conduct your own journaling exercises. Carve out some time during your retreat to focus on the goal that brought you to the retreat in the first place.

If you don't have a specific goal in mind, but still want to spend some time on self-development or life skills, here are some ideas.

THE LIFE AUDIT

This is where to start when you don't know where to start, when you aren't sure what your life's priorities are, or which direction you should be heading. Here are a few sources to check out prior to your retreat.

• Look for this book at your library: *The Life Audit* by Caroline Righton. The book contains many worksheets that help you figure out areas of your life that need your focus. Generally, the idea is that you take a look at different areas of your life – your health, relationships, image, finances, work, leisure, and community service – and take some time to decide what your idea of "perfect" would look like in each category. Next, you compare your reality with your idea of perfect. On a scale of 1-10, how close are you, for each category? Now review the 2 areas that got the lowest score. Which one is more important to you? And what is one thing you can do right now to get your closer to your perfect score? This book asks a lot of questions to guide you in your choices.

• Rating the different areas of your life is also known as the "wheel of life" exercise created by motivational speaker Zig Ziglar. You can access a free seven-page printable workbook at this website: TinyURL.com/ZigWheel.

• Alternatively, try the sticky note approach described at TinyURL.com/LifeAudit. Brainstorm and write down all your wishes, and then come up with a classification system for them – professional goals, personal goals, spiritual goals, etc. Is one pile a lot bigger than the others? Read the full post to see how the author categorized 121 goals by theme, timeframe, and other factors, to help reveal her life's priorities.

• If you don't want to make a to-do list, how about a to-stop-doing list? List the things you don't want to do anymore. Identify things you do that do not add value to your life; things that are time-suckers that don't actually make you happy. Consider the impact if you were to stop doing these things altogether.

• The 2-column approach: write a list of all the positive things that you do, and all the negative things. Things you think about. What you eat. What you read. What you watch. Who you spend time with. And then think really hard about the stuff that ends up in the negative column. Can you cut those things out completely?

OTHER SELF-DEVELOPMENT RESOURCES (THAT AREN'T AS BIG AS A LIFE AUDIT)

• *The annual review.* Sort of like a life audit, but with a spin. This is a review of the past 12 months and a plan for the next 12 months. Best-selling author Chris Guillebeau describes his annual review process at TinyURL.com/ReviewCG.

• Speaking of Chris Guillebeau, read *The Happiness of Pursuit*. In this book, he chronicles many folks who have adopted quests in their lives. He defines what he means by "quest" and shows the reader a fascinating viewpoint on the meaning of life.

• Create a vison board. When I first heard of vision boards, I thought the idea was stupid. I was taking Ali Edwards's *One Little Word* class, and she advised us to make a vision board for our words. My word was "fun". And like I said, I got the assignment and I thought, "how dumb." Then I realized that I didn't actually know what "fun" looked like to me. I sheepishly went over to Pinterest and typed in the word "fun" to see if anyone else knew what it looked like. After I created a Pinterest board of images that resonated with me, I used a Google Chrome extension called PinCo Collage (free) to create a digital vision board that I could download to my computer. PinCo Collage is really fun to use. It has some negative reviews, but it really is not difficult to use at all.

• If you like the kind of book that provides a different thought exercise every day for a year, try *Simple Abundance* by Sarah Ban Breathnach. Initially published in the early 1990s, it caught Oprah's attention and is still a top seller today. You should be able to easily find this in your local library. I believe Ms. Ban Breathnach is credited with creating the concept of the "gratitude journal." The thoughts and exercises are organized by calendar month. Try reading some of the essays for the current month during your spa retreat.

• If *Simple Abundance* is a little too frilly for you, try *Achieve Anything in Just One Year* by Jason Harvey. (Make sure to check the author's name

... there is more than one book with this title.) Although I find the title a little misleading, it's still an excellent resource containing 365 essays and action items for the reader. Check it out during your retreat and see if it is something you'd like to put in place for the next year.

• Another book with a somewhat misleading title is *Become An Idea Machine* by Claudia Altucher. This book gives 180 writing prompts – 6 months if done daily. Each prompt requires you to come up with a list of 10 things. For example, 10 ways you waste time every day, or 10 movies you love, and why. It's a challenge to the brain. It's usually easy to come up with 3 or 4 things, but 10 gives you a mental workout. Keep it up for 6 months, and Altucher promises you'll see improvements in your life simply because you've changed the way you approach problem-solving.

• If you like Excel spreadsheets and don't mind taking a look at your financial situation, here's a free link to help you outline your dreams, put a price on them, and then figure out how to make them happen financially. Uber-best-selling author and speaker Tim Ferriss (of *The 4-Hour Workweek* fame) provides an Excel spreadsheet that's kind of fun to play around with, especially if you have some disposable income. The link to his blog post about how to develop your own "dreamline" is at http://fourhourworkweek.com/lifestyle-costing/. From that page, click on "Dreamlining Calculators and Worksheet" and the Excel file will automatically download. You do not have to provide any personal information to get it. The blog post itself is a little sales-y, as of course he would like you to buy one of his books. But the short post contains good information, and if you are interested in reading more, you should easily find Tim Ferriss's books at your library.

• If the above actions feel too big for now, listen to Rachel Rofe's podcast episode called "How to feel more alive." This episode is only 8 minutes long. She provides encouragement and ideas for brainstorming a list of ideas for things that you enjoy doing, she says, "without turning it into a major life project." You can listen to the podcast directly from her website at TinyURL.com/RRAlive. Or if you just want to read a transcript, you can do that at TinyURL.com/AliveScript.

- Read *The Happiness Project* by Gretchen Rubin. Or, if you've already read it, try one of her two follow-up books. But really better than any of those is her podcast, *Happier with Gretchen Rubin*. Each episode is very enjoyable without getting into deep navel-gazing. Gretchen and her sister just talk happily and conversationally about the concepts presented in Gretchen's books, the science behind those concepts, and easy ways to incorporate happiness into your life. My only complaint about the podcast is the excessive use of sponsors for each short episode, but I just fast-forward through the ads.

- If you want to review other people's bucket lists for inspiration, check out Day Zero Project (https://dayzeroproject.com/ideas/). Look for the gray boxes with text. On the day I wrote this, a couple of the ideas were "learn how to make origami cranes" and "watch 10 movies that came out before I was born."

ENTERTAINMENT

Spa resorts typically offer some kind of evening entertainment, like live music. Make sure to schedule some kind of entertainment into your retreat. You could certainly head out to find some live music, or try one of the ideas below, which are more unique than what those resorts offer, anyway!

• Watch a movie that's outside your normal genre. You may discover something you really like. Seeing something new also exercises your brain. Or, watch the movie that your family keeps complaining about when you suggest it. You don't have to answer to anyone else during your retreat.

• Coloring books for grownups are trendy right now. Okay, a lot of people are making jokes about them. But they are fun. Just type in "coloring books" or "mandala" on Amazon.com and you'll get a lot of results with beautiful designs. Coloring books can help with relaxation or pushing you toward meditative moments. Or you can put on a podcast or some music while you color.

• Listen to comedy. On Pandora.com you can listen to jokes by famous comedians, for free.

• Or go to RadioLovers.com to listen to some old time radio. Choose from comedies, dramas, mysteries, big band, and many other varieties. You can listen directly from the website, or download specific episodes to play later.

• Gertrude Stein said, "Anywhere one lives is interesting and beautiful." Be a tourist in your own town. Seek out a new neighborhood to walk. Go to a popular destination that you've previously avoided. Look at restaurant reviews on Yelp and find something new that looks appealing. Visit one of the tiny museums or historical societies that no one ever sees. If you're staying in a hotel, pretend you are from out of town, and ask the concierge for recommendations for things to do and see. Travel awakens the mind. Pretend you are a traveler and view your town with new eyes.

• Perform a random act of kindness. If you have a little extra cash (even $10) try one of the Reddit "Random Acts" boards. The most popular are Random Acts of Pizza and Random Acts of Amazon. The Amazon one is really fun and does not require that you have a Reddit account to participate. (You'll need a Reddit logon for the pizza board, so you can send a private message to the pizza recipient to get their info.) On the Amazon board, you will find hundreds of user posts and very tiny text that says something like "http://amzn.com/w/xyz123". Copy and paste those links to a new browser tab and the user's wish list will open up. You can surprise people to your heart's content. Another way of doing this is by searching random names on Amazon (maybe a Facebook user that caught your attention) and seeing if you can find their wish lists. You can make up stories about how surprised they will be when they receive their gifts, especially if they weren't participating in the Reddit board or any other gift exchange.

• Read a book, just for fun. Re-read something you previously enjoyed. Or choose something from your stack of books you've been meaning to get to. Get ideas from WhatShouldIReadNext.com.

• If you're the kind of person who considers documentaries to be entertainment, especially if they are short, bring up some TED talks or try academicearth.org. The video electives on Academic Earth play in your browser and you don't have to create an account.

• Attend a one-day class. In your city, a number of classes may be available, such as cooking lessons, rock climbing classes, dance class, painting, etc. See what you can find that meets your interests and budget.

• Head out to wine bar and enjoy a glass of wine – either a favorite, or something new.

- Walk a labyrinth. Go to labyrinthlocator.com to see if there is a public labyrinth in your town. I tried the locator tool and was surprised that there actually is one in my small town, and I had no idea.

- Go geocaching. You used to need a handheld GPS device for this. But thanks to smartphones and the geocaching app (both iPhone and Android versions), you can now go treasure hunting more easily than ever.

- Learn a new skill or talent. You never know when you're going to find yourself in an impromptu talent competition. This happened to me at an amusement park once and all I could do on the spot was recite the list of linking verbs I memorized in 7th grade. I didn't win the contest. Don't let this to happen to you. Get prepared by browsing YouTube for dance moves you've always wanted to learn (Thriller, Saturday Night Fever, or the Dougie for example). Or check out WikiHow.com (login is not required) for things like How to Solve a Rubik's Cube, How To Whistle With Your Fingers, or How to Spin a Pencil Around Your Thumb. Learn a magic trick. Pick something like this, and then take a couple hours to practice, practice, practice.

- Spend a couple hours volunteering. If you plan ahead, you can schedule some time at a food bank or animal shelter. Or you can just go to a park or other public space and pick up trash. This may not quite be what people traditionally think of as entertainment, but service projects nearly always make the volunteer feel good.

SLEEP

Spa retreat hotels are places where the guest typically spends at least one night. Whether or not your personal staycation retreat includes an overnight stay, I encourage you to take this chapter very seriously and apply it to your everyday life. When you sleep less, you are less alive. When you are less alive, you are not the best version of yourself and you will achieve fewer goals. (Note: if you are sleep-deprived due to having a newborn in the house, please forget you read that last sentence. Instead, please know that your situation is temporary, and someday you all will be sleeping normally!)

In our culture, it seems there is a competition to see who can sleep the least. This attitude toward sleep is extremely unhealthy. At best, sleep deprivation affects your day-to-day quality of life in many ways (including impeding weight loss), and at worst, an increased mortality risk in those who consistently get less than 6-7 hours per night.

We are on the cusp of a sleep revolution, I believe. As the popularity of Fitbits, Apple watches, and similar wearable health monitoring devices increases, respect for sleep is going to finally reach viral public awareness.

Here are some ideas for making sleep an important part of both your retreat and your daily routine. Some of these activities are merely psychologically calming, while others have scientific backup. Consult your personal physician if you are taking any medications or if you have any concerns about trying these.

- Put your electronics in a timeout, preferably about 2 hours before bedtime. Read a paper book instead of looking at a screen.

- Enjoy some cinnamon milk. Warm a mug of milk on the stovetop or microwave until it is almost boiling (little bubbles around the edge). Remove from heat. Add 1 cinnamon stick, and then cover and allow to steep for about 10 minutes. (Put a lid on the pot, or put a plate or saucer on top of the mug.) Make sure to use a cinnamon stick, not powdered cinnamon. Drink, and enjoy. This remedy is only psychological. Although it is often reported to be a "proven" cure for insomnia, at this time there is no scientific evidence that cinnamon milk causes sleep. It is just a fun drink to make your spa retreat feel special and help you unwind before bed.

- Another beverage to try is tart cherry juice. Tart cherry juice is sold in grocery stores in the bottled fruit juice aisle. Look specifically for the words "tart cherry" or "Montmorency cherry." Some brands are 100 percent cherry juice, while others are a cherry/apple blend. There are a couple of scientific studies that indicate that drinking eight ounces of tart cherry juice (or juice blend) about one or two hours before bedtime will help cut down the time it takes to fall asleep. Montmorency cherries are known to contain melatonin, a hormone that aids in sleep, so it is assumed that the sleep benefit from the cherry juice is from the melatonin. (More research is still needed to prove the exact reason for the sleep benefit.) If you like cherry juice and you don't like swallowing melatonin pills, this is a nice treat before bed.

- Use one of the sources referenced in the meditation section of this book. They all have recordings specifically aimed at helping you sleep. There is a free sleep app called "iSleep Easy Free" that contains affirmations, breathing exercises, and a meditation specific for helping sleep. You might want to try this one. But in my opinion, the woman reading the affirmations and exercises on iSleep sounds utterly bored. (Maybe you prefer this when you trying to sleep.) If you are concerned about the light emitted from the screen interfering with your sleep, put your phone or tablet face-down.

- Cool your body. A drop in body temperature helps make you sleepy. Your body temperature drops after exiting a warm bath. Or you can just crank up the air conditioning in your room. If you want to take a bath before bed, experts say do it at least one hour before you plan to fall asleep.

• Play some white noise. If your mind races or you have tinnitus, white noise can be a sanity saver. White noise can be an electric fan, radio static, or a white noise machine or app.

• My personal favorite way to fall asleep is kind of controversial. I stream a TV show or movie on my phone, and I listen to it while I fall asleep. Many experts say that the light emitted from the phone is less than helpful, but it doesn't seem to bother me, though sometimes I do put my phone face-down. This method of falling asleep only helps me if the show/movie meets certain qualifications. It has to be a show I've seen before, and the show has to be nonviolent and have very little drama. I usually listen to *Friends* or *Parks and Recreation* on Netflix. This works for me because I force myself to listen to the dialogue instead of my own brain chatter. If the show has violence or drama, or if it's something I haven't seen before, it keeps me awake. As long as it's something sweet and benign, I'm usually asleep within 15 minutes. Science backs this up. You can turn off brain chatter in a matter of minutes simply by completely occupying your brain with something else.

• For a no-tech method, count your blessings instead of sheep, as the song says. Lie down, quiet your mind, and focus on listing everything you appreciate, however large or small.

WRAPPING IT ALL UP

At the close of your retreat, take a few minutes to jot down what went well, and what didn't. Think about your next retreat and schedule it right away. This is a habit that will serve you well for the rest of your life. I recommend taking personal retreats two to four times per year.

KEEP IN TOUCH

I would love to hear about your retreat. I also would enjoy helping you plan one, if you still suffer from "analysis paralysis" after reading this far. I collect sources for self-improvement, and not all of them made it into this book. Feel free to reach out to me if you have a specific issue you want to tackle. I may have an idea that would fit into your retreat. Also please feel free to contact me if you have any questions about how to use any of the sources I referenced. You can contact me at DIYSpaRetreat@gmail.com. Until then, please take care of yourself and have FUN!

APPENDIX

SAMPLE SCHEDULES

THE WEEKEND PERSONAL PLANNING RETREAT

Day One: Sleep as late as you want. No alarm clock is allowed. For breakfast, cook scrambled eggs, or order room service. Take a long shower or bath. Dress in comfortable clothes that make you feel good. Set the scene with candles, music, aromatherapy – whatever feels right to you. Sit on your bed or in a comfortable chair. Close your eyes, and meditate on your goals for the weekend. You have some planning to do, something that brought you to this retreat. Remind yourself of your reasons for being here. This may take five minutes, or twenty minutes. Just do this as long as you feel you need to. Next, think about your body from head to toe and consider whether you'd like to do any traditional spa beauty treatments. This is how I like to start my weekend retreat, and at a minimum I like to give myself a manicure. When I feel more "put together", I am better able to focus. You can do your own beauty treatments, or go out to a salon if you want to. Do this until lunch. Make your own lunch, or order food. After lunch, begin your focus on your personal planning goals. Set a timer for 45 minutes. Use one of the sources described in this book, or do whatever research you need to do to make your plans and decisions. When the timer goes off after 45 minutes, take a break for fifteen minutes. I like to do a yoga break. Yoga forces me to focus on nothing but the pose, or else I will tip over. This clears my mind from the previous 45 minutes. After the break, set the time for another 45 minutes and continue to work on your personal planning goals. When the timer goes off again, take another break. Then assess your progress and decide if you have met your planning goal, or if you need to continue tomorrow. You've done enough planning today. Prepare for dinner and some entertainment. Get ideas from the entertainment section of this book. Go to bed at a reasonable hour. This is very important to your physical and mental health. Use some of the tools described in the sleep section of this book.

Day Two: No alarm clock, unless you want one. Go out for a hike or nature walk. (Plan to have breakfast either before, or after, as your personal preference. Or perhaps both. I always enjoy Second Breakfast.) While you are hiking, allow your thoughts to return to your personal planning goals. Exercising makes the brain work in a different way than when you are just sitting at a desk. You may find that decisions come easier to you today, and especially while you are walking. When you return from your hike and have eaten a meal, consider whether you have met your goals for the weekend. If you have, then choose something from the entertainment section of this book. If you still have a decision to make or planning to do, then continue with the 45-minute timer method from yesterday. During the breaks, do something fun. Close your evening by watching a movie – either an old favorite, or something that's been on your list for a long time.

THE RELAXING BUT NOT-TOO-LAZY RETREAT

This is the retreat where you want to take some time for yourself, but don't want to get too contemplative. You don't have any big decisions or resolutions to make, but you're also thinking that if you're going to take time away from your family, it better be worth it. Consider scheduling some volunteer hours into this type of retreat.

If you know you are regularly sleep-deprived, then do sleep as late as you want. Have breakfast, then go out for a nature hike. This is good for your body and your mind as well. When you return, choose to do one of those things that you just never get to during your regular day. This could be something like a haircut, or a stack of books you've been meaning to finish. Resist the urge to tackle a to-do list. Focus on things that make you feel good. In the evening, go out and be a tourist in your own town. Visit a restaurant or venue that you've never been to before. Help other tourists by writing a Yelp review of the place you just visited.

THE DISTRACTION RETREAT

Schedule this type of retreat when you need a respite from your everyday life. This is a good one for caregivers who can have a nurse or partner replace them for the day. (Make sure you know why you are choosing distraction and that it is a safe and healthy response to your situation.)

If at all possible, check into a hotel. If you have a Netflix account, bring your laptop (make sure the hotel has reliable Wi-Fi). Watch movies from your queue, or binge-watch a TV show. If you don't use Netflix, then just enjoy the hotel TV. Use their pay-per-view service to watch the latest movie, and order room service at the same time. Take a long bath while listening to upbeat music. Then repeat. I don't recommend yoga or meditation during this type of retreat, only because your thoughts may return to the very things from which you are taking a mental break.

THE RETREAT AT A PARK OR BEACH

Choose books to read or media to listen to. If you want to listen to audiobooks, podcasts, etc., download them before you go. Don't forget your headphones. Pack a picnic lunch, pick one up at the store, or have a friend or loved one pack a special surprise picnic for you. Bring a blanket or towel. Drive to a park or beach. This could be a favorite spot, or one you've never been to before. Then just enjoy everything you packed, at your leisure. Stay out until it gets dark. You could do this one in a library as well (minus the picnic), if the weather isn't working out.

THE CHRISTMAS PLANNING RETREAT

I like to do my holiday planning retreat-style. I get it all done in one fun personal day, and I feel a lot more organized through the holiday season. Otherwise, I find myself planning menus, gift ideas, etc. on the fly and it feels a lot more hectic.

Put on Christmas music, if you like. Then begin by asking yourself what your goals are for the holiday season. What does the holiday mean to you? A time to reconnect with family? A time for religious reflection? A time for traditions? If you've never really asked yourself these questions, take as much time as you need to answer them honestly. Are there things you have been doing every year out of habit, and not because you actually want to? Break from your old traditions. Plan a holiday that is enjoyable for you and your family, filled with events that you really love. Work on a budget, a gift recipient list, and a gift idea list. Do you plan to make any gifts? Plan out a schedule, and give yourself a date upon which you will give yourself permission to abandon any unfinished crafts and go out and purchase gifts. Will you travel? Will you be hosting guests? Work on travel arrangements. Write down the favorite holiday foods that you and your family enjoy. Plan meals and grocery lists. Find those old recipes. Schedule volunteer work and service projects. Research concerts or other events that that you would like to put on your family's calendar. When you're done outlining your plan, sit back and enjoy a Christmas movie.

Spa Meal Recipes

Coconut Honey Granola

Source: SpaIndex.com: Guide to Spas (Reprinted with permission)

Dry Ingredients
- 3 cups rolled oats (not instant)
- 1 cup wheat germ
- 1/2 cup chopped almonds
- 1/2 cup pepita seeds (roasted pumpkin)
- 1 cup shredded, unsweetened coconut

Wet Ingredients
- 1/4 cup oil
- 3/4 cup honey
- 1 teaspoon vanilla extract

Directions

1. Mix all dry ingredients in a deep bowl.
2. Mix all wet ingredients in a small bowl.
3. Warm the wet ingredients *slightly* in your microwave to make pouring easy.
4. Pour the warmed wet ingredients over the dry ingredients, and toss to "dress" the granola.
5. Spread the granola 1/2 inch deep on a lightly oiled cookie sheet, lightly oiled.
6. Bake at 250 degrees F for 30 to 45 minutes until golden brown.
7. Check it and stir occasionally during this period, as the sides and bottom brown first.
8. Let cool, and stir while cooling.
9. Store in airtight container.

Asian Slaw

Adapted from The Pampered Chef

For the salad

- 16-oz package of cabbage slaw or broccoli slaw
- 2 red apples, chopped
- 4 green onions with tops, sliced
- ½ cup peanuts
- Cooked chicken, optional

For the dressing

- 3 Tbsp cider vinegar
- 2 Tbsp water
- 1 Tbsp vegetable oil
- ¼ cup sugar
- 1 clove garlic, pressed

Directions

1. Mix all the salad ingredients together in a large bowl.
2. Mix all the dressing ingredients together in a small bowl.
3. Pour dressing over salad, and toss to coat. I like to make my salad in a large bowl that has a lid, if possible. Then I can just put the lid on the big bowl and shake it up.

Grilled Caprese Sandwich

Ingredients

- 2 slices sourdough bread

- Butter

- Pesto (from a jar – I don't bother making from scratch)

- 1 tomato, sliced (or try with sliced apple or mushrooms, if you prefer)

- 2 slices mozzarella cheese, or handful of shredded mozzarella. Or provolone slices. Whatever you have.

Directions

I like to make this on a large griddle, so I have more room to work. But if you don't have a griddle, just use a big frying pan. Heat the griddle or pan on medium-high, while you butter both sides of both pieces of bread. Then put both pieces of bread on the griddle/pan, and brown them. Once browned, flip them over. Immediately put your cheese on one of the pieces of bread, so it can start melting. Turn down the heat to low. Carefully spread some pesto on the other slice of bread on the griddle. Put sliced tomatoes (or apple or mushroom) on top of the melted cheese. After the bottom of the bread has browned, remove to plate, sandwich the 2 pieces together, and enjoy.

Spa Water Recipes

Cucumber Water (blended)

Blend all of the following ingredients together: 1 cucumber, peeled and cut into cubes, 3 tablespoons lemon juice, 5 cups water, and ¼ cup sugar. Ready to drink immediately. Pour over ice, if you like.

Cinnamon Water

You need to plan ahead for this one. Make the water the night before you plan to drink it. Simply put some cinnamon sticks (3-5) in a pitcher of water. Voila, in the morning you have cinnamon water. This is one of my favorites!

Ginger Pineapple Water

Here's another one to make the night before. Combine the following in a 2-liter pitcher: 3 cups of fresh pineapple, 5 fresh slices of ginger, 1 sliced lime, a dozen mint leaves, ½ teaspoon salt, then top off with water. Allow the flavors to infuse in the refrigerator for several hours.

Watermelon Basil Water

One more that needs to be made in advance. Combine the following in a 2-liter pitcher: 3 cups cubed watermelon, 6 basil leaves (or more, if you love basil), ½ teaspoon salt, then top off with water. Allow the flavors to infuse in the refrigerator for several hours.

Mango Blueberry Coconut Water (blended)

Combine the following in a blender: 3 cups coconut water, 1 cup plain water, 1 cup blueberries, 1 mango (seeded), 1/8 teaspoon salt. Ready to drink as-is, or pour over ice.

Raspberry Lime Sparkling Water

Combine the following in a pitcher: 2 cups raspberries (muddled if fresh, thawed if frozen), juice of one lime, 5 cups sparkling water. Pour over ice and enjoy.

Strawberry Peach Sparkling Water

Combine the following in a pitcher: 1 cup strawberries, 2 cups peach slices, 5 cups sparkling water. Pour over ice and enjoy.

Affirmations

I have enough. I am enough. My ordinary self is enough.

Peace, love, and joy abide in me.

Inhale the future, exhale the past.

I am me, and I am amazing. (Or, in the words of Dr. Seuss, "There is no one alive who is Youer than You.")

I am capable and deserving of success. I am just as capable and deserving as anyone else.

I will change only what I have the power to change. I accept the things I cannot change.

(Inhale) I love ... (exhale) myself

Good is good enough.

SUGGESTED SPA MUSIC

I found that if I simply did a search for "meditation" playlists, a lot of the music sounded too sad. Here are my recommendations for music that's not depressing, that you can play in the background.

Search your favorite streaming music player (Spotify, Amazon Music) for the word "baroque." Or Bach. Usually these won't let you down. I like the album *Baroque Masterpieces* by Neville Marriner. It is available on Spotify.

Amazon Music (Amazon Prime) has an album called "Spa Music Collection" that is nice, if you like flutes and water sounds. I also like the collection called Meditation: Classical Relaxation.

On Pandora, try creating a station based on one of the following key words: Karunesh (Zen Breakfast), Cirque du Soleil, or Calm Meditation. If you don't have a paid subscription to Pandora, I recommend activating your free trial just before your spa retreat. I find the advertisements too distracting during a retreat. I really like my Cirque du Soleil station because the music is upbeat, but the lyrics aren't in English, so I'm able to focus on my projects more easily.

If you want a more modern sound for your ambient music, try the "Chill" channel on Apple Music. It's in the Electronic category.

YouTube is also a great source for background music or nature sounds. One more plug for TheHonestGuys.

30 ADDITIONAL IDEAS TO TURN THE DIY SPA RETREAT INTO A COUPLE'S RETREAT

If you'd like to turn your DIY Spa Retreat into a couple's retreat, that's easily done.

Volunteering, touring your own town, cooking, hiking, geocaching, the life audit, vision boards, random acts of kindness, taking a class together...nearly all of the activities referenced in The DIY Spa Retreat can be customized for couples.

Here are 30 additional suggestions to consider adding to your couple's retreat. Just as I recommend for a personal planning retreat, make sure you know the goals of your couple's retreat before you decide on your activities. If your retreat is of a more serious nature, you might not want to do #22 (hotel with waterpark). If your retreat is one of community service, check out #26-30. And if you're looking to have some fun and strengthen your relationship, then read on...

1. Meditate together. Choose a guided meditation that makes sense for you as a couple. You can start your practice during your retreat, and then discuss whether it makes sense in your everyday schedules to continue meditating together going forward. After the meditation, talk to each other about your experiences. Close the session by facing each other and looking into each other's eyes for at least one minute. It will feel awkward at first, and giggling is fine. However, you may find that this one action is very powerful for your relationship, so give it a chance.

2. Take a road trip for the weekend, or even for just one day. Being trapped in the car together, away from your everyday

lives, can help push your relationship to a new level. Or maybe I'm just saying that because my honeymoon with my husband was a 3-week road trip. We had been a couple for years before our wedding, but we both agreed that we felt closer after our road trip.

3. If you have a pickup truck, throw all your blankets and pillows into the back and drive out at night to do some stargazing.

4. Have a no-tech day. This is probably more beneficial in a couple's retreat than in a solo personal planning retreat. Turn off the devices and really be together now.

5. Make a bucket list or date night idea list together. Maybe add an element of surprise by writing your ideas on craft sticks or little paper scrolls stored in a mason jar. When you're ready for an adventure, pull one out at random.

6. Play your favorite songs for each other. Listen to each song in full. Afterward, explain to your partner why the song means so much to you. Then let your partner do the same. Make sure to actively listen to your partner.

7. Or, go to a local art museum and do a similar exercise. Each partner chooses a favorite piece of art, and then explains what makes it so meaningful.

8. Consider starting a marriage journal or appreciation journal. My opinion is that this really works best when both partners are on board with the idea, so don't push your partner to agree to it. You can use journal prompts like: "Remember when…", or "You are amazing because…" Or come up with your own rules for how the journal is to be used. Maybe one partner takes it for a week, then the other partner gets the journal the next week, and so on.

9. Couples yoga. Yes, it's a thing. I hesitated to mention it because

it kind of makes me want to gag. Go on Pinterest and type in "couples yoga". There's something really #humblebrag about it, right? BUT, if you're really fit and gorgeous and maybe want to hire a photographer to show everyone how fit and gorgeous you are, go for it. It's technically called Acro Yoga.

10. Write a mission statement for your relationship or your family.

11. Drag out the fondue pot or get one from the thrift store. Fondue isn't so much fun on a solo retreat, but great for couples!

12. Go rock climbing. Or maybe just to a rock climbing gym. You can spot each other. A trust exercise and physical exercise, all in one!

13. Rent a tandem bike. You know, the bicycle built for two. Take turns sitting in the front seat.

14. Look through your wedding album, or watch your wedding video.

15. Put on some music and do a jigsaw puzzle together.

16. Find the tallest building in your town. Head to the roof or highest floor to see the sunset. Or if you live in a hilly town, find the highest hill.

17. Re-create your first date.

18. Play Top Chef and challenge each other. Go to the grocery store and split up. Each partner chooses three items. Meet up again at the checkstand with your surprises, and then go home and see what you can cook up. You may want to set some ground rules first, like, "nothing gross" or "nothing too passive-aggressive" or "nothing you know I'm allergic to!"

19. Photograph each other.

20. Do this totally cool bookstore date. http://loveactually-blog.blogspot.com/2009/05/bookstore-date.html

21. Eat spaghetti while watching Lady and the Tramp.

22. Consider booking your retreat at one of those hotels that has an indoor waterpark.

23. Go to your local science museum and build something together.

24. No science museum? Build a house of cards.

25. Launch a new blog together. Just for fun. Do not try to monetize it.

26. Put away all the carts in a grocery store parking lot.

27. Go to a drive-through and pay for the car behind you.

28. Write a note to a military serviceperson who is deployed.

29. Put together a care package for the homeless.

30. Plan a party together, for a friend's or relative's birthday.

ABOUT THE AUTHOR

Heather Tremko is a collector of information. She's an avid reader, podcast junkie, and fan of the Oxford comma. She filters through the zillions of bits of data out there, and brings back only the best free or frugal tools to help you live your best life.

Heather knows what it's like to live a hectic life. She's blessed with two young, energetic, and very loud daughters. As a new mother, she juggled parenthood and a full-time job, all the while trying to maintain self-care. She also supported the family while her husband was attending nurse practitioner school. Talk about stress! She believes that it is critical for each of us to take time for ourselves in order to maintain our sanity. For Heather, learning to take care of herself was vital.

The knowledge she gained while learning to care for herself led Heather to write her first book, The DIY Spa Retreat. She believes that you don't need to spend hundreds or even thousands of dollars on a spa day when you can create your own special and highly customized spa day for a lot less. Heather maintains balance and peace in her life by frequently treating herself to her very own DIY retreats. You can do the same!

Heather lives in Oregon with her husband and two wonderful children.

Printed in Great Britain
by Amazon